HOW TO MANAGE SOCIETAL CONSEQUENCES OF STEROIDS

ESSENTIAL STEPS TO CURTAIL STEROID ABUSE

JORDAN HAVENSTRITE

TABLE OF CONTENTS

ESSENTIAL STEPS TO CURTAIL STEROID ABUSE________________1

INTRODUCTION________________2

CHAPTER ONE________________3

WHAT ARE STEROIDS?________________3

CHAPTER TWO________________10

What are steroid injections and how are they used?________10

CHAPTER THREE________22

How can we curtail their abuse?________22

CHAPTER FOUR________24

Management Strategies and Supporting Evidence________24

CHAPTER FIVE________27

Areas of Uncertainty________27

CONCLUSION________________29

COPYRIGHT PAGE

All rights reserved. No part of this publication may be republished in any form or by any means, including photocopying, scanning, or otherwise without prior written permission to the copyright holder.

Copyright ©2022 JORDAN HAVENSTRITE

INTRODUCTION

Steroids are synthetic versions of hormone-like substances produced naturally by the human body. Steroids are made to operate similarly to these hormones to lessen inflammation.

They go by the name corticosteroids and are distinct from the anabolic steroids used by athletes and bodybuilders. Steroids are excellent at lowering inflammation and will help with symptoms like swelling, pain, and stiffness but they won't heal your ailment.

In most cases, the body's natural response to an infection or bacterial growth is inflammation. To combat infections or bacteria, your immune system creates more fluid, which results in swelling, redness, and heat in the affected area. If you've ever suffered a skin injury like a cut or wound, you could have observed this.

In some cases, including rheumatoid arthritis, the immune system unintentionally causes inflammation in the joints or other regions of the body, which if unchecked can result in lasting damage. To lessen this immunological response, steroids can be given.

This page is about steroids that can be taken as tablets, liquids, creams and eye drops, and ointments. Information about **steroid injections** is covered on a different page.

This page discusses several forms of steroids, including tablets, liquids, creams, eye drops, and ointments. On a distinct page, information about steroid injections is presented.

There are various ways to use steroids.

CHAPTER ONE
What are steroids?

Are there any reasons why I won't be prescribed steroids?

If you have an infection or any open sores on your body, you might not be able to start steroids since they could prevent these conditions from healing or mask some of your symptoms.

Diabetes, heart or blood pressure concerns, as well as mental health conditions, may all be impacted by steroids. The person who is treating you must ensure that the steroids aren't exacerbating any existing conditions if you have any of them.

Prednisolone may not be safe for you to take if you have systemic sclerosis since it can harm your kidneys at certain doses.

If you have a skin infection, you won't be able to use steroid creams or gels. If you have any of these illnesses, you might not be able to use steroid creams. Other skin conditions like rosacea, acne and ulcers can also be aggravated by steroid creams.

You may need to refrain from wearing contact lenses while receiving treatment with steroid eye drops if you typically wear them.

How are they taken?

Depending on the disease you have, there are several ways to take steroids and different dosages may be necessary. You can get an indication of how frequently you would need to take steroids from the table below.

Always take your medications exactly as your doctor has instructed.

Tablets, liquids, and soluble tablets

• Typically once each day.

• Ideally early in the day.

• Before or after eating to avoid gastrointestinal issues.

Creams and gels
• For a few weeks, typically once or twice every day. Your doctor might advise taking them for a longer amount of time but less frequently.

• Should only be applied to skin that is damaged.

Eye drops and ointments
Usually one drop in each eye each time you take it; • May need to be taken repeatedly throughout the day.

To lessen the chance of side effects, the lowest dose for the shortest amount of time will be administered to you. As your symptoms go better, your dose will likely be progressively decreased, or your doctor may recommend a medicine with lower potency.

You must first speak with the healthcare provider before stopping your steroid use.

If you stop taking steroid pills abruptly after using them for more than a few days, you may experience withdrawal symptoms as a side effect. To make sure your symptoms don't come back, you can receive a little dose for a long time, sometimes known as a maintenance dose.

Side-effects and risks
Some patients will experience side effects, as with all medications. If you take steroids frequently or at a high dosage, these side effects are more likely to occur.

To keep your condition under control, the person who is treating you will make sure you are taking the lowest dose possible. To protect your stomach, your doctor may also prescribe a medication known as a proton pump inhibitor or another treatment.

The following list of steroid side effects includes some of them:

Tablets, liquids, and soluble tablets
• gaining weight and having a greater appetite;

• experiencing heartburn, indigestion, or stomach pain;

- having trouble sleeping;

- changing one's attitude;

- bruising easily;

- having stretch marks.

Creams and gels

Stretch marks, changes in skin tone, thinner skin, stinging or burning where the cream has been administered, and increased hair growth are all possible side effects.

Eye drops and ointments

- burning or stinging after applying drops to the eyes

- a peculiar aftertaste from ingesting drops.

Steroid therapy may alter your mood; you can experience extreme highs or lows. People with a history of mood disorders may experience this more frequently. Talk to the doctor who is prescribing you steroids if you have concerns about this.

Long-term steroid use increases your risk of contracting infections. It's vital to let your doctor or the rheumatology nurse know right away if you experience any new symptoms after starting steroids, such as a fever or malaise.

If you get chickenpox, shingles, measles, or if you come into touch with someone who does, go see your doctor or the person who is treating you right away. People who take steroids occasionally get severe cases of these disorders, and it may take additional treatments before you begin to feel better.

Long-term usage of steroids can weaken your muscles and occasionally interfere with a woman's menstrual cycle.

Other complications

Although steroid creams and eye drops often don't have major adverse effects, if you use them frequently or in large doses, the medicine may enter your bloodstream and raise your risk of

Error! No text of specified style in document.

experiencing side symptoms that are typically reserved for steroid pills.

You'll occasionally have your blood pressure and blood sugar levels examined because steroids can occasionally influence diabetes, high blood pressure, or epilepsy. If necessary, the healthcare provider may adjust the dosage of your drugs.

In individuals without a history of diabetes or high blood sugar, steroids can occasionally result in these conditions.

Steroids may have an impact on the eyes, worsening glaucoma or producing cataracts, for example. Serous chorioretinopathy, also known as core-ee-oh-ret-in-op-ath-ee, is an eye condition that develops when fluid builds up in a particular area of the eye. Be sure to notify your doctor right away if you experience any vision changes, such as hazy vision.

Cushing's syndrome is a different ailment that drugs can occasionally cause. This can result in skin thinning, stretch marks, and a rounder face, but after steroids are discontinued, it normally goes away.

Steroid use in children and teenagers can occasionally delay growth, thus it's important to frequently measure their height. They might be referred to a specialist doctor for advice if their growth slows down.

Managing side effects

It's crucial to monitor your weight while taking steroids because they can make you gain weight or have a stronger appetite. You should be able to prevent gaining weight by choosing wholesome foods and including moderate amounts of physical activity in your daily routine.

The use of steroids may weaken bones, which may result in osteoporosis. Your chances of breaking a bone increase if you have this condition, often even after very slight falls or bumps.

To assist prevent this, your doctor could suggest that you take bisphosphonate medications, calcium supplements, and vitamin D in addition to the steroids. Regular exercise, especially activities

Error! No text of specified style in document.

like walking that need your bones to support the weight of your body, can also help lower the risk.risk of developing osteoporosis.

Along with avoiding smoking and excessive alcohol consumption, you should make sure your diet has enough calcium.

Effects on other treatments

It is possible to take steroids with other medications. However, because some medications may interact with steroids, you should speak to your doctor before starting any new ones, and you should let anyone else who is treating you know what medications you are taking.

Avoid using over-the-counter medications or herbal supplements without first seeing your physician, rheumatology nurse, or pharmacist.

Let your doctor know if you're taking any of the following medications because some of them may interact with steroids:

• blood thinners or anticoagulants like warfarin;

• medications for epilepsy like phenytoin or carbamazepine;

• medications for diabetes;

• the prostate cancer medication Xofigo.

Vaccinations

Live vaccines, including yellow fever, may need to be avoided if you're taking steroid tablets. When a live vaccine is required, your doctor will go over the potential dangers and advantages with you. Whether you need the immunization also depends on the dosage of steroids you're taking.

It is acceptable to receive vaccines if you are using a steroid cream, but you must advise the person administering the injection to avoid the area being treated with the cream.

If you take only a small amount of steroids, you might be able to receive the live shingles vaccine (Zostavax). You could also be able to receive the non-live shingles vaccination (Shingrix) as an alternative. Your medical group will be able to offer advice in this regard.

Error! No text of specified style in document.

Since they are not live vaccinations, the annual flu shot and the immunization against the most prevalent cause of pneumonia do not interact with steroid pills. To lessen your risk of contracting certain infections, you must have these immunizations.

Having an operation

You may have to stop taking steroids if you are undergoing surgery. However, don't do this without first consulting your doctor or surgeon, since you may be able to continue taking them in some circumstances and may need to have your dose adjusted **before** the operation.

The choice will be made based on how long you've been taking them, the dosage, and the area of your body that needs surgery.

Alcohol

Your stomach may become irritated if you consume alcohol or steroid pills. Reduce your alcohol consumption if you experience indigestion or other stomach issues after starting steroids because alcohol is likely to make things worse.

A weekly intake of 14 units of alcohol is the maximum recommended amount in the UK. Instead of saving up these units to consume all at once, spread them out over the week and have some days without alcohol.

Fertility, pregnancy, and breastfeeding

Prednisolone is among the steroid tablets that, according to current recommendations, can be taken while pregnant. They are frequently used to treat flare-ups in expectant mothers.

It's crucial that a mother stays well during pregnancy and that flare-ups are avoided, so if you're thinking about starting a family, you should talk about this with your doctor. Do not stop taking steroids before consulting your doctor if you become pregnant while taking them.

The guidelines state that adults can breastfeed while taking steroid pills even though small levels of steroids may transfer into breast milk. No research has demonstrated that this is hazardous to your baby. If you have any questions, talk to your doctor about the dangers.

While steroid creams are acceptable to use while pregnant, you'll need to be careful to clean off any cream before nursing. During pregnancy and breastfeeding, extremely potent topical steroids are typically not recommended.

CHAPTER TWO
What are steroid injections and how are they used?

The human body naturally produces certain steroids. Artificial steroids have similar anti-inflammatory effects to real steroids.

They differ from the anabolic steroids that bodybuilders use to bulk up and strengthen their muscles.

For the treatment of arthritis and related disorders, steroids can be injected directly into the afflicted area or consumed as tablets.

People with rheumatoid arthritis and other forms of inflammatory arthritis are frequently advised to receive steroid injections. They might also be suggested if you have osteoarthritis and your joints hurt a lot or if you temporarily require more pain relief. Pain should be reduced as a result of the injection's potential to reduce inflammation.

Steroid injections can address the symptoms of your problem but not the underlying cause.

Uses

For injection, a variety of steroids are available. Hydrocortisone (hi-dro-cor-tee-zone), triamcinolone (try-am-sin-o-lone), and methylprednisolone are three common steroid injections (meth-al-pred-niss-o-lone).

The effects of some steroid injections should continue for approximately a week and begin to reduce pain within hours. These short-acting soluble steroids may be referred to as such by your doctor or another healthcare provider. When medicine is soluble, it immediately dissolves in your body and begins to work.

Other steroid injections take about a week to start working, but they can relieve your symptoms for up to two months. Because the drug needs more time to enter your system, these are referred to as less soluble.

Your condition will also influence how quickly and how long the medication takes to take effect.

All ages of patients, including kids and teenagers with juvenile idiopathic arthritis, can receive steroid injections (JIA).

However, young patients should utilize steroid injections cautiously. The shortest amount of time at the lowest possible dose should be administered. Children who receive excessive steroid therapy risk having their growth hampered.

How is it taken?

You will discuss the best steroid combination and dosage for you with your doctor or nurse. Depending on your health and symptoms, this will vary.

Before your first injection, they might want to check your blood pressure and blood sugar levels as steroid injections might cause these to rise. If either is raised, they might postpone the injection.

Steroids can be injected depending on where the pain and inflammation are:

An intra-articular injection goes directly into an inflammatory joint; a peri-articular injection goes into the soft tissue next to the joint.

Intramuscularly, which is the term for injection into a muscle.

Most injections may be done quickly and easily. They will be performed by a medical expert in a hospital, clinic, or doctor's office.

An ultrasound scan may be required to locate the area of inflammation so that the steroid can be injected precisely and effectively. An ultrasonic scan produces an image of a portion of the inside of a body using high-frequency sound waves. Numerous injections can be administered without using ultrasonography.To lessen the pain of the injection, a local anesthetic may occasionally be administered together with the steroid. This would imply that your pain would disappear in a matter of minutes. Unless you've been given a long-acting local anesthetic, the effects of a local anesthetic can subside in as little as 30 minutes. The anesthetic may cause some numbness in you, which could continue for up to 24 hours.

If you're getting a steroid injection, loose-fitting clothing might be more comfortable.

Following your steroid injection, you might be instructed to wait for 10 to 15 minutes in the clinic. It would be beneficial to be near medical personnel if you do experience any sort of injectable reaction.

If you plan to have a local anesthetic, you may want to organize transportation home following the injection because driving may be challenging while you are numb.

Steroid injections are frequently helpful in the short term for some illnesses, such as inflammatory kinds of arthritis, while you and your doctor look for the best medications to control your arthritis over the long run. In this situation, the need for injections should decrease once your arthritis is under good control.

Is there anything else I need to know before I have a steroid injection?

If you have an infection, especially one that is in the area of your body that requires treatment, you will not be able to have a steroid injection.

Because receiving a steroid injection can cause your blood sugar levels to rise for a few days following the injection, if you have diabetes, you should talk to your doctor or another healthcare provider about this. Following a steroid injection, you need to keep an eye on your blood sugar levels.

There is proof that administering too many steroid injections to the same place can harm internal tissue.Your doctor will likely advise against receiving more than three steroid injections into the same area of the body i12 assessed. Depending on your symptoms, you might be advised to consume less than that.

You should talk to your doctor if you have hemophilia (he-mer-fill-ee-ur), a disorder in which your blood doesn't clot properly, as you may be more susceptible to bleeding into the joint.

For the first two weeks following a steroid injection, moderation is key. A tiny chance exists that overusing a joint just after

Error! No text of specified style in document.

receiving a steroid injection could harm the tendon. Following this point, it's critical to keep up with any exercises your healthcare provider has recommended. slowly build up your activity levels.

Your physiotherapist will assist you in striking the ideal balance between rest and exercise if you are receiving physiotherapy.

Side-effects and risks

In most cases, steroid injections have no negative side effects. While they may feel a bit uneasy during the injection, many people believe that this is not as unpleasant as they had anticipated.

Occasionally, within the first 24 hours following injection, people experience an increase in their joint discomfort. It normally goes away on its own in a few days, but paracetamol or other over-the-counter pain relievers can be helpful.

With harsher mixes, methylprednisolone, and triamcinolone, the risk of adverse effects is highest.

The skin at the injection site may occasionally shrink or change color as a result of injections, especially the stronger ones.

Rarely, you can develop an infection in the joint where the injection was administered. See your doctor right away if your joint starts to hurt more and get hot, especially if you're feeling sick.

The potential for further steroid-related side effects, like weight gain, frequently worries people. When compared to tablets, one benefit of steroid injections is that the dose may frequently be maintained low. This indicates that these additional side effects are quite uncommon unless injections are administered often, more frequently than a few times per year.

Period alterations in women can occasionally result from steroid doses. People's moods can also vary as a result; you might experience extreme highs or lows. If you've previously experienced mood disorders, this might be more likely. Please speak with your doctor if you have any concerns.

Error! No text of specified style in document.

Can I take other medicines along with steroid injections?

Along with steroid injections, you can take other medications. To ensure that your blood is not too thin for the injection, you might require an additional blood test if you use an anticoagulant, such as warfarin, a medication that thins the blood. This is due to the potential for joint hemorrhage.

You should let the person administering the injection know that you take anticoagulants. Before receiving the steroid injection, your warfarin dosage may need to be adjusted.

Vaccinations

In the near term, the impact on your body's immune system is lessened by steroid injections. They do this to lessen inflammation.

Some vaccinations operate by inoculating you with a tiny amount of a specific disease so that you develop immunity to it. A steroid injection won't be permitted very soon after receiving certain immunizations. If you recently received a vaccination or are scheduled to receive one soon, discuss when you will be able to have a steroid injection with your healthcare provider.

Fertility, pregnancy, and breastfeeding

According to current recommendations, steroid use during pregnancy **or breastfeeding** is safe. Single steroid injections are safe for use during pregnancy, lactation, and fertility, and they can be **an** effective therapy in these circumstances. However, before receiving a steroid injection, you should discuss it with your doctor if you're expecting or nursing.

Steroid Side Effects: How to Reduce Drug Side Effects of Corticosteroids

How to approach the advice listed below: You should talk to your doctor about any of these recommendations that are unclear to you or that you believe might not apply to you. Also, keep in mind that the dosage and duration of steroid use have a significant impact on adverse effects. If you take a low dose, your risk of experiencing major adverse effects is very low, especially if you take the precautions we'll cover below. You might start to feel uneasy about taking steroids after reading about these negative

Error! No text of specified style in document.

effects. Before beginning these medications, you should be fully aware of the hazards. But rest assured that many people take steroids without experiencing any or only slight negative effects. Please keep in mind that steroids can frequently be incredibly effective and even save lives. Please review any of the advice given here with your doctor if it is unclear to you or appears unrelated.

Please take note of the "steroids" we are referring to Anti-inflammatory steroids (corticosteroids) like prednisone, methylprednisolone (Medrol®), and dexamethasone (Decadron®) are referred to as "steroids" in this context. The following does not apply to anabolic or "androgenic" steroids (such as testosterone), which have some chemical similarities to anti-inflammatory steroids but act very differently.

Understanding corticosteroid side effects

Corticosteroids may cause any of the following negative effects when used over an extended **pad** But by adopting the precautions we'll talk about below, you might be able to lower the dangers.

Increased doses needed for physical stress

Your body's capacity to react to physical stress can be decreased by using steroids for longer than two weeks. When under extreme stress, such as after surgery, significant dental work, or a serious infection, a greater dose of steroids may be required. This can be required for up to a year after you stop using steroids.

Talk about this possibility with the doctor, dentist, or whoever is currently caring for you. If your doctor or surgeon is aware that you have been taking corticosteroids, they can keep an eye on you more closely following surgery even if they don't believe you need to take the additional steroid at the time of operation.

Steroid withdrawal syndrome

Our adrenal gland, which creates our body's steroid hormones, can be slow to produce steroid hormones when anti-inflammatory steroids have been taken for a while and then abruptly stopped. The intricate process that our body uses to produce the anti-inflammatory steroid hormone may be inhibited as a result of taking anti-inflammatory steroids (cortisol). The hypothalamus and pituitary gland, which are all involved in the process of stimulating the adrenal gland to produce cortisol, can be

Error! No text of specified style in document.

suppressed by these anti-inflammatory chemicals. For instance, the generation of ACTH by the pituitary gland, which stimulates the adrenal gland to produce cortisol, can be suppressed. The adrenal gland's capacity to produce cortisol can also exhibit some suppression.

Rapid steroid withdrawal may result in a condition that includes weariness, joint discomfort, stiffness, tenderness, and fever. It could be challenging to distinguish these symptoms from those of your underlying illness. Some of these symptoms are still possible even with the gradual withdrawal of steroids, albeit typically in weaker forms.

Rapid steroid withdrawal can occasionally result in a more serious syndrome of adrenal insufficiency. Blood pressure dips and chemical changes in the blood, such as excessive potassium or low sodium levels, might result from this, along with other symptoms and health issues. Sometimes an operation or an injury can trigger this. Because of this, it's important to always let your doctors know if you've received steroid treatment in the past, especially within the last year, so they can watch out for the emergence of adrenal insufficiency during situations like surgery.

• If you experience any of these symptoms while tapering off steroids, talk to your doctor. Depending on how you are doing, your doctor will work with you to gradually reduce your steroid dosage at a safe rate. Ask your doctor if it's possible to reduce your steroid dosage at each visit.

• Keep in mind that you still need to taper off of steroids gradually even if you are experiencing an adverse effect from them.

• In general, quicker tapering of steroids is possible when taken for less than two weeks.

Infection

Steroid use over a long period can reduce your immune system's capacity to fight infection and raise your chance of getting sick.

• For as long as you are on steroids, you should get an annual flu shot because steroids can lower your immunity to infection. Discuss the potential of receiving "Pneumovax," a vaccination against a specific form of pneumonia, as well as "Prevnar 13," another pneumonia vaccine, with your doctor if you take steroids for a longer period. Another option to consider is the Shingrix® vaccine for shingles. Your doctor will decide which immunizations you require after considering your age and risk factors.

• Patients should seek immediate medical assistance if they exhibit symptoms of a potential infection including a high temperature, a productive cough, pain when urinating, or huge "boils" on the skin. If you have a history of tuberculosis, have been exposed to it, or have had a positive tuberculosis skin test, inform your doctor about this.

Gastrointestinal symptoms

When taken with NSAIDs like ibuprofen or aspirin, non-steroidal anti-inflammatory medicines (NSAIDs) like steroids may raise your risk of stomach ulcers or gastrointestinal bleeding. If at all feasible, avoid mixing NSAIDs and steroids. While taking prednisone, your doctor may want you to continue taking low-dose aspirin, but they may also consider adding a prescription for stomach protection while on steroids.

• Stools that are dark or tarry or that are persistently severe should be reported to your doctor.

• To help reduce stomach irritation, take the prescribed steroid alongside antacids or just after a hearty meal. Steroids may make you more ravenous.

Osteoporosis

Osteopenia and osteoporosis are two conditions that can result after medication, which can also raise the risk of bone fractures. Many patients will be requested to undergo a bone density test at

Error! No text of specified style in document.

the beginning or before their steroid medication, particularly if the steroid dose is high. If the density is low, a follow-up bone density study will be done to evaluate how well the steps you will take to stop bone loss are working. A person can lose 10% to 20% of their bone mass within the first six months of corticosteroid therapy, therefore prevention measures are crucial.

• The majority of people on corticosteroids will need to take a calcium supplement if they don't consume enough calcium naturally (if possible, this is the best option). For information on how much calcium you need for your age and sex and how to get it as much as you can from food, see this National Institutes of Health reference.

• The majority of persons using corticosteroids should consume 800 international units (UI) of vitamin D per day, which is the recommended minimum daily intake. If you require a greater dose of vitamin D, your doctor may check your level.

Limiting alcohol use and smoking lowers the risk of osteoporosis.

Exercise that involves bearing weight, such as walking, running, dancing, etc., helps maintain bone mass.

• Alendronate (Fosamax®), Prolia®, and other drugs may be prescribed to those taking corticosteroids who have low bone density.

• Evaluate the chance of falling. Make a complete inspection of your home and address any issues that could lead to a fall, such as installing night lights and removing scatter rugs from the path between the bedroom and bathroom.

Weight gain

Your metabolism and how your body stores fat are both impacted by steroids. This may make you hungrier, which could result in weight gain and, in particular, more fat deposits in your abdomen.

Track your caloric intake and engage in regular exercise to try to avoid gaining too much weight. But avoid letting weight increase

Error! No text of specified style in document.

undermine your self-worth. Be aware that in the six to a year after you stop taking steroids, losing weight will be simpler.

Insomnia

Steroids may make it difficult for you to fall asleep, especially if you take them in the evening.

If at all possible, the doctor will try to have you take the complete recommended daily dosage in the morning. If you do this, you might get a better night's sleep (evening doses sometimes make it difficult to fall asleep).

Mood changes

Your mood may be impacted by steroids, particularly when taking daily amounts of more than 30 mg. Some people may experience intense "up" feelings or depression for no obvious reason. Simply being aware that steroids occasionally have this effect makes it less of an issue. In certain cases, this adverse effect necessitates a reduction in the steroid dosage. When steroids are required, a different medicine may occasionally be administered to deal with the mood issue. Ensure that your family is aware of this potential adverse effect.

Sometimes, it helps just to be aware that steroid use can impact your mood. But occasionally, this effect will call for a reduction in the steroid dosage. Another drug may occasionally be added to the steroid regimen if keeping the same dosage is required to treat the mood disorder.

Make sure your loved ones are aware of this potential side effect so that if you react to them in strange ways, they will understand what's going on. For them to assist you in identifying any behavioral changes, it is ideal to inform your family and friends about this potential side effect as soon as you begin the medicine.

Fluid retention and elevated blood pressure

These medications can encourage fluid retention and occasionally cause or exacerbate high blood pressure since cortisone is

Error! No text of specified style in document.

involved in regulating the body's balance of water, salt, and other electrolytes.

• Keep an eye out for any ankle swelling and let your doctor know. Diuretics are beneficial for occasional patients (water pills). A low-sodium diet can help manage blood pressure and prevent fluid retention.

• If you have a history of high blood pressure, get your blood pressure checked frequently while you are using steroids. Some patients' blood pressure may rise as a result of steroids.

Elevated blood sugar

Long-term usage of cortisone may result in high blood sugar levels or possibly diabetes since it helps to maintain normal levels of glucose (sugar) in the blood.

• If you have diabetes or are taking corticosteroids, you should monitor your blood sugar levels while you are taking them.

Eye problems

Sometimes, steroids might lead to glaucoma or cataracts (increased pressure in the eye).

•

If you have a history of glaucoma or cataracts, keep a watchful eye on your eye health while taking steroids. You must visit an ophthalmologist if you experience any visual issues while using steroids. When taking corticosteroids, temporary blurred vision is frequently not a serious issue; nevertheless, if you suffer other, new visual symptoms while taking the medication, it is always advisable to schedule an appointment with an ophthalmologist.

Atherosclerosis (hardening of the arteries)

The rate of "hardening of the arteries" may accelerate as a result of steroids, raising the risk of heart disease. If steroids are taken for a long period and at large doses, the risk is likely to be significantly greater.

• A low-cholesterol diet might be beneficial. If you have symptoms of a cardiac condition, such as chest pain, seek medical help right away. Discuss any cardiac risks with your doctor, such as those

Error! No text of specified style in document.

related to activity, weight, and cholesterol levels, that can be changed.

Aseptic necrosis

• Aseptic necrosis, which is bone deterioration caused by steroids, can occur when they are used for extended periods and at larger doses (also known as osteonecrosis or avascular necrosis). Although it can occur in other joints as well, hip problems are the most frequent.

When Should You Call a Doctor for Steroid Addiction?

It is reasonable for parents to ask their healthcare practitioner for assistance if they have concerns that their child may be abusing anabolic steroids. Counseling for mental health issues is also appropriate.

What Tests Confirm Steroid Abuse?

Steroids frequently stay in the body for lengthy periods and can be found in urine drug tests. Because they are designed to be harder to detect, some designer steroid medicines may evade detection. The World Anti-Doping Agency, however, collaborates with numerous labs to create tests that enhance the detection of performance-enhancing drugs in the body.

Sometimes medicines employed as masking agents are discovered even though the steroid itself is not. Water tablets or diuretics bumetanide and furosemide may result in a false-negative test. The presence of these masking substances in a urine sample is also regarded as a failed test for professional and elite athletes.

What Is the Treatment for Steroid Addiction?

• Those who use anabolic steroids don't experience the same level of addiction as those who abuse alcohol or other narcotics. However, some research points to the possibility of steroid demands that are comparable to caffeine cravings.

• In terms of the related lifestyle and the pursuit of the effects that anabolic steroid use results in, it is addictive. This includes concerns about one's perception as well as the truth of gaining muscle and growing larger. To address the underlying problems that caused the first steroid use, counseling may be required.

Error! No text of specified style in document.

Counseling may be helpful if there are psychological adverse effects as well.

Error! No text of specified style in document.

CHAPTER THREE
How can we curtail their abuse?

Education on the hazardous side effects and signs of misuse is the most crucial factor in reducing abuse. The ability to excel in sports and have fantastic bodies without using drugs must be understood by athletes and others. They should prioritize eating well, getting enough sleep, and maintaining good general mental and physical health. All of these things affect how the body is built and trained. Without using steroids, millions of people have achieved athletic success and great looks.

Path to improved safety

Steroids are powerful, life-saving medications. They may, however, also have negative side effects. These include weak bones, dry mouth, irregular menstrual periods, and thin skin. They may raise your blood pressure or blood sugar levels. The short-term usage of steroids is frequently recommended due to these negative effects.

Your body produces steroids on its own spontaneously. Your body produces more steroids when it is under stress, such as after an infection or surgery. Your body may cease producing its steroids if you take steroid pills, sprays, or lotions. If you consistently take steroids, it

 is possible that your body won't produce enough of them while you're under stress. You might need to take more steroid medication if this occurs.

Reduce the dosage of steroids you take gradually by **a** little over time. You'll be given a regiment for taking the medication from your doctor. You must carefully adhere to this schedule. The doctor will order you to cease taking steroids after the dose has sufficiently decreased. Without consulting your doctor beforehand, do not reduce or stop taking the medication.

Your body may take longer than usual to produce the additional steroids you require if you stop using them. A quick blood test to check on your body's health may be recommended by your doctor. They may ask you to start or resume taking your steroid medication if necessary.

Error! No text of specified style in document.

Things to consider

Your body may need a few weeks or months to naturally produce more steroids. You can have steroid withdrawal symptoms at this time. These include experiencing faintness, wooziness, or fatigue. Body aches and stomach pain could be present. If you experience any unusual symptoms in addition to these, speak with your doctor.

There are a few safe ways to discontinue using steroid medications. These products may also lessen the effects of steroid withdrawal.

• Unless your doctor instructs you to, do not stop taking your steroid medication.

• Avoid using any other medications while using steroids without first consulting your doctor. This covers both prescription and over-the-counter medications.

• Tell your doctor straight away if you feel ill while taking less steroid medication.

• Think about purchasing a bracelet that includes your medical information. This wristband will alert medical personnel that you take steroids if you go unconscious. Never fail to disclose to medical staff that you are using steroid medication.

CHAPTER FOUR
Management Strategies and Supporting Evidence
Start an Immunomodulator (Azathioprine or 6-Mercaptopurine)

The thiopurine analogs that have been used to treat IBD for more than 30 years are related to azathioprine (AZA) and 6-mercaptopurine (6MP). Some studies indicate that AZA is steroid-sparing in UC, even though the evidence for the use of immunomodulator therapy in Crohn's disease is stronger than in UC. AZA at a dose range from 1.5 to 2.5 mg/day for 6 months dramatically lessens steroid dependence, according to two randomized placebo-controlled trials published more than 20 years ago and one published just last year. The most recent of these 3 trials defined steroid dependence as needing 10 mg/day of steroids throughout the previous 6 months with at least 2 attempts to stop taking the medicine. This patient's scenario closely matches this criterion. In that trial, 6 months following study enrollment, 53% of steroid-dependent patients who were randomly assigned to receive AZA (2 mg per kilogram per day) were in remission and no longer taking steroids. In comparison to the placebo group, this was statistically better since 21% of steroid-dependent patients who got 5-aminosalicylate therapy (3.2 g/day) simultaneously went into remission and stopped using steroids.

Immunomodulators should be used chronically to lower the chance of relapse, therefore problems with long-term usage, notably infections, cancer, and pregnancy, are especially important for this patient. The usage of AZA/6MP raises concerns that lymphoma risk will grow. In IBD patients taking AZA/6MP, a recent meta-analysis projected a 4-fold increase in lymphoma. Despite this purportedly elevated risk, it is thought that immunomodulator therapy is generally more beneficial than harmful. As a result, IBD treatment treatments have been accepted by AZA and 6MP. The usage of AZA and 6MP may expose the fetus to danger. Category D pregnancy medicines according to the Food and Drug Administration (FDA) include AZA and 6-MP (evidence of fetal risk but benefits to mother might outweigh potential risk). These medications are frequently used during pregnancy to keep the mother in remission despite

Error! No text of specified style in document.

this FDA classification.This justification is supported by extensive knowledge of the use of these drugs in pregnant transplant patients, a growing body of data demonstrating their safety in IBD, and the significance of administering these drugs to keep the mother well and in remission during the pregnancy. There is currently no convincing evidence that the prevalence of congenital abnormalities among offspring of women exposed to 6MP/AZA has increased. The immunomodulator methotrexate, which is used to effectively treat active Crohn's disease, is noteworthy since it is contraindicated during pregnancy (category X) and is ineffective for treating UC.

Start Biologic Therapy (Infliximab)

A chimeric monoclonal antibody called infliximab is directed against the pro-inflammatory cytokine TNF-alpha. Since 1998 and since 2005, infliximab has been licensed for the treatment of UC and Crohn's disease, respectively. The results of the first five controlled trial trials examining the effectiveness of infliximab for the treatment of UC were mixed. However, infliximab consistently showed to be beneficial for the treatment of UC in the 2 most recent big randomized controlled trials, the Active Ulcerative Colitis Trials (ACT) I and II. Patients who failed medical therapy with >20 mg/day of steroids, AZA, or mesalamine (ACT II only) when they flared on a lower dose of prednisone qualified as steroid-dependent patients under the inclusion criteria for ACT I/II. 20% to 25% of all patients who were randomly assigned to an induction regimen of 5 mg/kg of infliximab at 0, 2, and 6 weeks, followed by a maintenance dose every 8 weeks, were in remission and off corticosteroids at week 30 even though data for the steroid-dependent subgroup were not reported separately (7 months). In the placebo group, 3%–10% of patients were in remission and not taking steroids at the same time. This was significantly superior to that group. Similar to purine analogs, infliximab is advised for long-term use to lower the chance of recurrence. Infliximab chronic use is also advised to limit the emergence of drug-related antibodies, infusion responses, and diminished drug efficacy. When used to treat various disease states, infliximab has been linked to an increased risk of infection and cancer. In ACT I and II studies, there were no lymphomas recorded at 1 year, which is relevant to the risk of

Error! No text of specified style in document.

malignancy associated with prolonged treatment. To fully evaluate this risk with prolonged usage, however, long-term cohort studies and post-marketing surveillance on a larger group of UC patients would be necessary. Infliximab is a medication for pregnancy classified by the FDA as having a category B risk to the fetus (either animal studies have not demonstrated a fetal risk but there are no controlled studies in pregnant women or animal studies have shown an adverse effect that was not confirmed in women in the first trimester). A small but rising body of research points to infliximab's minimal risk during pregnancy. The substance does pass through the placenta and can be found in the child up to six months after birth.

Proceed to Surgery (Proctocolectomy J Pouch Ileoanal Anastomosis)

Surgery has always been regarded as the only method of UC treatment because it is 100 percent effective. UC surgical therapy has developed through time, much as UC medical therapy. Young individuals are frequently given a proctocolectomy with ileal pouch-anal anastomosis (IPAA) as an alternative to the conventional permanent (Brooke) ileostomy. Total proctocolectomy with IPAA can, in the hands of a skilled surgeon, lead to low complication rates, positive functional results, and better quality of life (QOL), albeit the improvement in QOL, is greatly influenced by QOL before surgery. Nevertheless, IPAA is a technically challenging procedure with a 5%–18% risk of pelvic abscess and short-term pouch leakage. The risk of developing cancer after surgery is very minimal if the rectum is entirely removed along with the colon. Rare reports of malignancy in the pouch and the remaining rectal cuff have been documented. Therefore, when considering pouch surgery, the function of the pouch and fertility is more important long-term consequences for the majority of patients to address. 9% to 20% of operations are known to have chronic pouchitis. Between 2% and 10% of pouches fail after a year. Patients often have 6 bowel motions every day (1 nocturnal). About 7% and 12% of people experience incontinence during the day and at night, respectively. A recent meta-analysis revealed a threefold rise in infertility following pouch surgery. Based on seven studies, medication treatment for UC resulted in a weighted average infertility rate of 15% while

Error! No text of specified style in document.

pouch surgery resulted in a weighted average infertility rate of 48%. Patients may still become pregnant with medical aid. It is thought that pelvic adhesions and scarring are to blame for the loss of the capacity to conceive.

Error! No text of specified style in document.

Azathioprine or 6-Mercaptopurine for Steroid-Dependent Ulcerative Colitis

There hasn't been a controlled trial of 6MP in UC. AZA and 6MP are regarded as interchangeable in the treatment of UC, nevertheless, they are related substances. AZA and 6MP are equally effective in treating Crohn's disease if the correct target dose is met and enough time is given for the therapeutic benefit to materialize. AZA and 6MP both have a target therapeutic dose of between 2-3 mg/kg and between 1-1.5 mg/kg, respectively. AZA and 6MP's therapeutic effects can take up to 17 weeks (4 months) to manifest.

What is the Optimal Strategy for Starting Azathiopurine/6-Mercaptopurine?

Leukopenia and abnormal aminotransferase levels would be minimized while the time to the therapeutic benefit of commencing AZA/6MP was sped up. Starting AZA/6MP at the intended dose and keeping an eye on the outcomes of laboratory tests has been one approach. A second approach has been to begin administering AZA/6MP at a low dose and increase it to the target dose while keeping track of the outcomes of laboratory tests. A third approach has been to base the initial dose of AZA/6MP on whether thiopurine methyltransferase (TPMT), the enzyme that converts AZA/6MP to inactive metabolites, is active normally, intermediately, or inactively. Unfortunately, no thorough research has been done to determine which of these tactics is better. It should be highlighted that despite the third strategy's rising popularity, monitoring blood tests is still necessary because leukopenia can occur even with normal TPMT levels. Only one-fourth of actual cases of leukopeniaaaresare linked to the existence of TPMT genetic polymorphism.

Step-up, Top-down, or Combination Therapy for Steroid-Dependent Ulcerative Colitis?

For this patient with steroid-dependent UC, there are no head-to-head studies to compare the efficacy of starting AZA versus 6MP (step-up), infliximab (top-down), or both (combination therapy). In a current clinical trial for Crohn's disease, patients who were randomized to receive AZA, infliximab, or combination therapy and who were unexperienced with both biologic and immunomodulator therapy and needed frequent corticosteroid administration were assessed for rates of steroid-free remission at 6 months.

Should Patients on Long-Term Infliximab Also Be on Long-Term Azathiopurine/6-Mercaptopurine?

In addition to infliximab, patients are frequently given either AZA or 6MP to lower the likelihood of infliximab-neutralizing antibodies. More recently, the risk of malignancy (hepatosplenic T-cell lymphoma) with combined immunosuppressive therapy has encouraged some specialists to stop administering AZA/6MP to patients receiving infliximab after six months or to substitute low-dose methotrexate. In steroid-dependent UC, the benefits and drawbacks of this practice pattern have not yet undergone a thorough analysis.

Error! No text of specified style in document.

CONCLUSION
WHY YOU SHOULD NOT SUDDENLY STOP TAKING STEROIDS?

It is VERY essential to take each dose as prescribed for steroid treatments lasting more than a few days, and you should only discontinue taking them under a doctor's supervision. This is because your body quits producing enough steroids to maintain essential processes after a few days or weeks of steroid use (such as blood pressure). A sudden stop from taking medicine could result in a rapid drop in blood pressure and have an impact on blood sugar levels. To give your adrenal glands enough time to resume producing their steroid hormones, you will need to "taper" (gradually reduce) the amount.

In most cases, people who have taken steroids for less than three weeks won't need to "taper," but you should always speak with your IBD team before ending medication.

Sadly, occasionally when people go back on their steroid dosage, their IBD symptoms come back (known as steroid dependence). If this occurs, other medications, such as azathioprine, may be suggested to help you completely taper off steroids.

Error! No text of specified style in document.

9 798353 452980